Angel, Blessing, Crippled, the ABCs Of One Child's Story

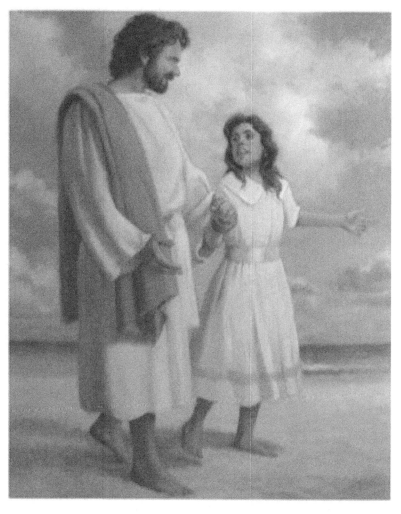

By
Dr. Linda Nell Drake Coakley

Kristy is an Angel

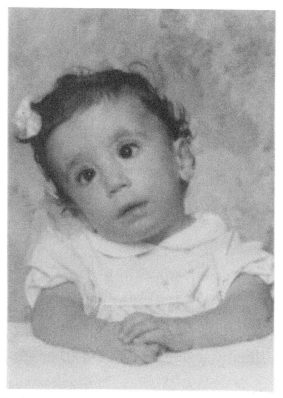

Kristy Marie is an angel, a precious blessing from God.
Living with Kristy is like living with an angel.
She exhibits a sweet, graceful presence and consistent
kindness. Even her movements are angelic. She extends her
arms outward as if they are wings and she is about to fly.

Kristy grows sweeter every day of her life, bearing great
affliction with grace and beauty.

Kristy was age 6 months in the picture on this page.

Walking with God

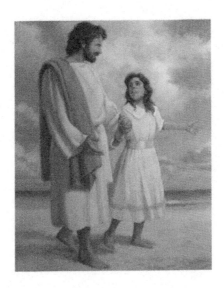

Kristy is a crippled child and cannot physically walk or talk yet she has spiritually walked with God all her days.

Kristy was age 15 when this portrait was painted. The original painting by Mitch Mann hangs in our living room at home to inspire Kristy and to assure her that Jesus is with her.

I believe Jesus is holding her hand throughout her very precious life. He holds her right hand saying,

Fear Not, I will help you, Isaiah 41:13.

Kristy is a Blessing
Not a Burden

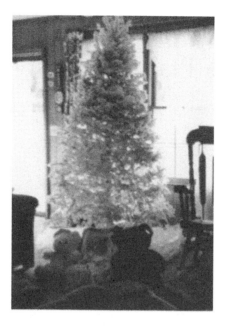

Kristy is in her baby carrier under the Christmas tree that first day with us.

Like all good and special blessings, Kristy was a heavenly gift from above. She blessed our lives from the start, coming to live with us as a foster child at age 4 months. Kristy was admitted to Vanderbilt hospital at age 5 weeks to undergo open-heart surgery.

After 2 months in the neonatal intensive care and the hospital, Kristy struggled in and out of several foster homes as a very fragile child with her many medical challenges. Weighing only 11 pounds when she came to us, Kristy tried to smile, but could not. She held her right arm close to her body and had difficulty breathing. She had a large pink birthmark (angel kiss) over most of her face that faded by age 2.

A Place for Kristy

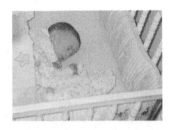

Above and beyond her physical challenges was a lovely person shining through, a beautiful sweet little girl. Her eyes, from day 1, pleaded, "keep me." And one day on the way home, I looked at Kristy in her infant seat and promised her that I would keep her as long as I could. With God's help, I have been able to keep that promise. God had prepared a place for Kristy in our home, but most importantly, in our hearts.

Taking care of Kristy was one of the greatest challenges of my life. There were many dark days with little sleep, no rest, and serious illnesses when Kristy was close to death. Only God's strength enabled me so that I could have done all that I have done for this sweet little girl.

I'm so thankful that He loved her through me. I feel so honored to have known her and to have been in His presence with Kristy. What a tremendous blessing she has been to my life!

Kristy was Crippled Physically
Yet she was a Perfect Person

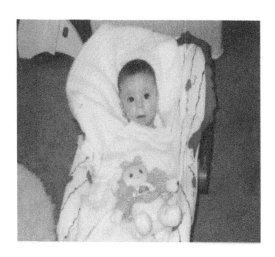

From the day Kristy was born in Baptist Hospital on
August 23, 1994, suffering was part of her life. It
seemed that each trip to the physician or hospital
revealed another diagnosis. As a person, Kristy was
perfect.
Sweetness and integrity were evident from the start.

Many visits to emergency rooms, clinics, medical supply
companies, pharmacies, the pediatrician, neurologist,
orthopedic and cardiac surgeon, cardiologist,
pulmonologist, ophthalmologist, otolaryngologist,
dermatologist, dentist, developmental and genetics
clinic, early intervention center, physical therapists,
occupational therapists, speech therapists, children's
services, medical day care, the school system, home
health services, and respite services are some of the
resources necessary to provide care and help for Kristy
and children like Kristy who are disabled.

Physical Challenges

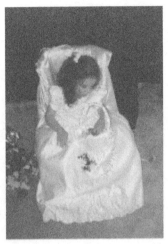

Kristy was diagnosed with Fetal Alcohol Syndrome. Septal defects of the heart are associated with Fetal Alcohol Syndrome. Kristy was found to have congestive heart failure due to the septal defect and that is why she had to undergo open-heart surgery at age 5 weeks.

She came to live at my home as a foster child on December 30, 1994. Little did anyone know how great and extensive would be Kristy's affliction. Kristy's MRI revealed thin brain structures. Later, a CT scan showed that her corpus callosum, the part of the brain that facilitates communication between the hemispheres, was missing. There was retarded growth of the brain and overall growth. All these problems are also part of the spectrum disorder that is Fetal Alcohol Syndrome. Later diagnosed with cerebral palsy, failure to thrive, global developmental delay, scoliosis, asthma, restrictive airway disease, Kristy lived as a medically fragile child, susceptible to many illnesses and frequent infections that resulted in frequent hospitalizations.

Who Made the Afflicted?

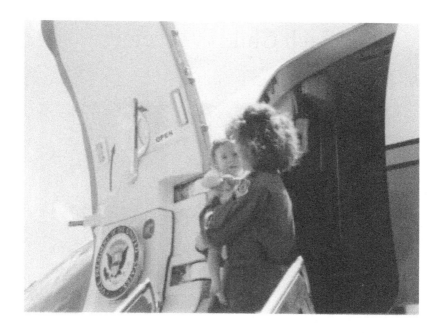

Kristy on steps of Air Force II in the arms of
adoptive mom, Captain Linda Coakley

Throughout the ages mankind has pondered issues related to
human suffering. Great philosophers and simple children
look on the afflicted with disturbed wonder. What
happened? Why did this happen? Who made this person like
they are?

The answer is in God's Word in Exodus 4:11.

> *Who has made man's mouth? Or who makes the
> mute, the deaf, the seeing or the blind?
> Have not I, the Lord?*

> Proverbs 22:2 *Jehovah is the maker of them all.*

Each Child is Precious

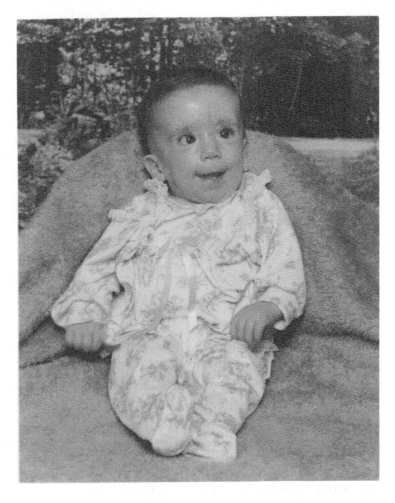

Kristy had great difficulty seeing due to severe strabismus (crossed eyes), repaired by surgical correction at age 2 at Vanderbilt Hospital.
Strabismus is one aspect of Fetal Alcohol Syndrome.

The Lord Makes all Things and
The Lord Made Kristy

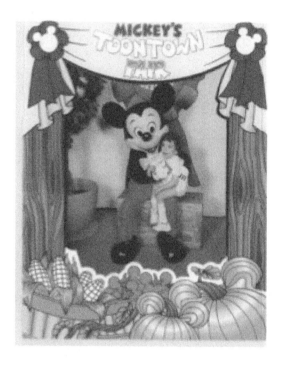

Psalms 119:73 *Thy hands made me and fashioned me.*

Isaiah 43:7 *I created him for my glory, I have formed him; yea, I have made him.*

Isaiah 44:1-2 *Yet hear now, O Jacob My servant, and Israel whom I have chosen. Thus says the Lord Who made you and formed you from the womb, I will help you.*

Isaiah 44:24 *Thus says the Lord, your Redeemer, And He Who formed you from the womb: I am the Lord, Who makes all things.*

Bless the Afflicted
and You Bless Jesus

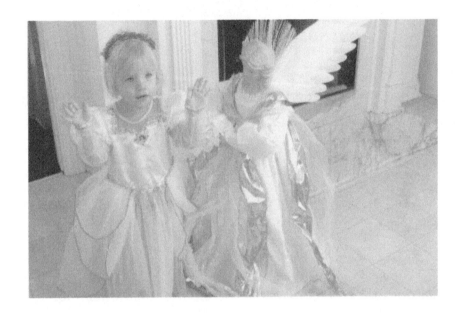

Emma Grace is my granddaughter. Emma has been a great blessing to Kristy. Kristy's eyes light up whenever I say, Emma Grace. Kristy smiles or laughs when Emma talks to her on the phone. When Emma comes to visit, she dances for Kristy to lift her spirits. She says, "I love you, Kristy Boo" (Emma's nick name for Kristy).

Matthew 25:40 Jesus said, *If ye have done it unto one of the least of these, Ye have done it unto me.*

Pray for the Afflicted

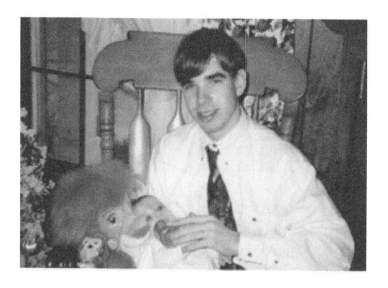

My son, Eddie, prays for Kristy. Eddie is a minister and the members of his church, Trinity Baptist in Cayce, SC, also pray for Kristy.

Eddie was only 17 when Kristy came to live with us. He was a senior in high school and had already been called by God to preach the gospel.

He was so wonderful and accepting of Kristy into our home.

Why Doesn't God Heal the Afflicted?

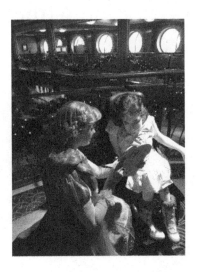

Up most every night caring for Kristy with her many medical problems I worried about waking and disturbing Eddie. Kristy's needs were so great. Eddie never complained but said, "What a sweet thing to give your life to."

James 5:14-15 *Is any among you sick? Let him call for the elders of the church; and let them pray over him, anointing him with oil in the name of the Lord: and the prayer of faith shall save him that is sick, and the Lord shall raise him up . . .*

Yes, Kristy has been greatly prayed for. We prayed that she would walk and talk. Why God heals some and not others is hard to understand and perhaps only in heaven will such deep questions be answered. Several people including myself dreamed of Kristy walking. I know she will walk and talk in heaven one day. What a day that will be!

Included

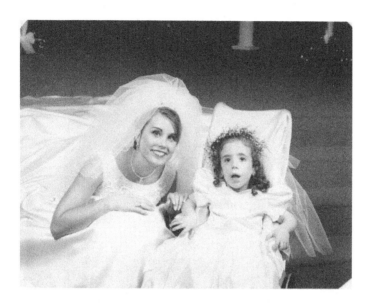

Kelly, my daughter-in-law, included Kristy in her wedding as the flower girl. Could you somehow include a disabled person in your life? Inclusion is therapeutic and enhances self-esteem and the quality of life.

Not long ago tears came to the eyes of one of our neighbors who said that she still remembers how little Kristy looked in her wheel chair coming down the aisle at the wedding. Little Kristy cannot walk or talk or do any of the activities of daily living that most people take for granted yet she has blessed, impacted, and inspired so many lives!

How can anyone question the sanctity of each life? Each person is a unique human being created in God's image.

Inclusion principle: Include the poor, The lame, the maimed, and the blind and You will be blessed

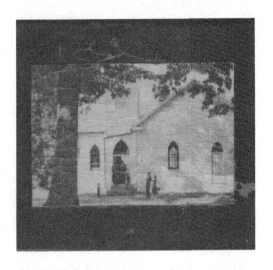

Throughout Kristy's life she demonstrated joy in going to church. There have been several Sunday-School teachers and other volunteers of different churches through the years who have greatly blessed Kristy. There is however only one church that Kristy has attended all her life, the Battle Creek Baptist Church. The members there have welcomed Kristy to their fellowship. They pray for her and list her name on their prayer roster. The youth of the church have blessed Kristy with gifts that they made for her. The members show the compassion of Christ toward Kristy.

Would it not be wonderful if like Battle Creek, the whole world would practice inclusion of the afflicted!

Biblical Story of Inclusion

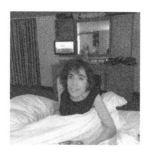

There are many beautiful stories in the Bible of inclusion, of how God notices and lifts up the lowly. Jesus's mother, Mary, magnified the Lord with these words found in Luke 2:52-53: *He hath put down princes from their thrones, And exhalted them of low degree. The hungry he hath filled with good things; And the rich He hath sent empty away.*

Luke 14:12-13 *When you give a dinner or supper, do not ask your friends, your brothers, your relatives, nor your rich neighbors, . . . but when you give a feast invite the poor, the maimed, the lame and the blind, And you will be blessed, because they cannot repay you; for you shall be repaid at the resurrection of the just.*

There follows the story of a man who prepared a great supper and was offended when those he invited refused the invitation. These are the orders he then gave his servant found in Luke 14:21, 23 *Go out quickly into the streets and lanes of the city and bring in here the poor, and the maimed, and the lame, and the blind . . . and compel them to come in that my house may be filled.*

Inclusion of the afflicted persons of the world is important. Remember that each of us is at God's mercy to be included in the kingdom of heaven. The verses above promise you will be repaid one day for inclusion of those who cannot repay you now.

Who Sinned?
Kristy's Afflictions are not Her Fault

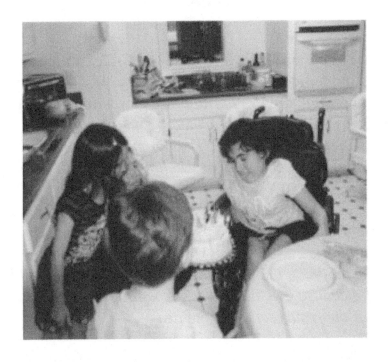

John 9:1-3 *Now as Jesus passed by, He saw a man who was blind from birth. And his disciples asked Him, saying, "Rabbi, who sinned, this man or his parents, that he was born blind?" Jesus answered, "Neither this man nor his parents sinned, but that the works of God should be revealed in him.*

This story relieves a great burden from those who are already burdened by affliction. Afflictions are not punishment for sin. Their lives bring glory to God and inspire us all.

Hope for the Afflicted and the Outcast

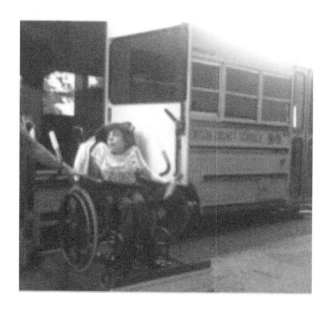

Micah 4:6-7 *In that day says the Lord, I will assemble the lame, I will gather the outcast and those whom I have afflicted; I will make the lame a remnant and the outcast a strong nation; So the Lord will reign over them in Mount Zion From now on, even forever.*

What a beautiful picture painted by this passage, of the Lord gathering the afflicted to Himself in Mount Zion.

God Hears Their Cry
and Pleads Their Cause

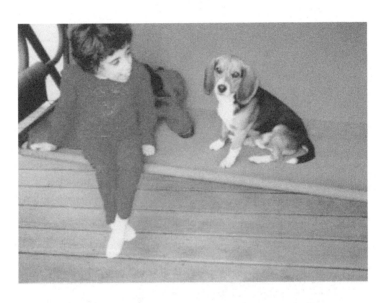

Kristy loved her dog, Copper and the story he was named
after, Disney's Fox and the Hound

Psalms 22:24
*For He has not despised nor abhorred the affliction of
the afflicted;*
Nor has He hidden His face from Him
But when He cried to Him, He heard.

This verse gives comfort not only to the afflicted, but to
their mothers, fathers, and others who so grieve for
them and whose utmost concern is that there will be
someone to care for their afflicted child when they can
no longer do so.

Proverbs 22:22-23 *Neither oppress the afflicted in the
gate; For Jehovah will plead their cause, And despoil
of life those that despoil them.*

Sure Promise
God will not Forget the Needy

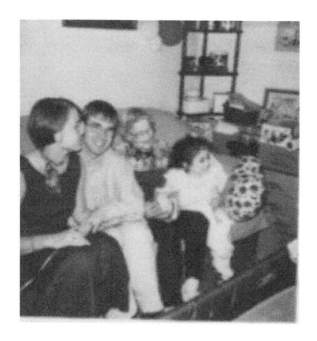

Kristy with Grannie Drake, Eddie and Kelly

2 Kings 20:5
I have heard your prayer, I have seen your tears; surely I
will heal you.

Psalms 9:18
For the needy shall not always be forgotten;
The expectation of the poor shall not perish forever.
God has not forgotten the afflicted.

Grannie Drake's Loving Message

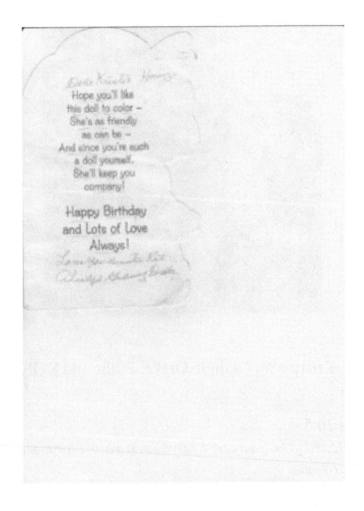

This card is from my mother. She and Daddy loved Kristy and Mama called her, Grannie's Baby.

Kristy's Grandparents

Mama and Daddy set beautiful examples of love and nurturing. Mama had 14 brothers and sisters and Daddy had 9. There were many nieces, nephews, cousins, 5 children, and 15 grandchildren. Our home was always full of happy family and friends. Mama cooked great meals, sewed clothes, soothed hurts and cared for the sick taking in those with hard times. Mama and Daddy welcomed everyone.

Mama and Daddy were very poor yet always treated each who came for help as a person of worth. They were giving and loving, always helping and welcoming neighbors and family. Daddy raised a garden every year and shared all that he had giving vegetables to any and all who needed help or who just came to visit.

Mama had many cats, dogs, and chickens out in the yard of our country home. Whenever one of the animals was blind or lame, Mama sheltered them and gave extra care and concern. Mama and Daddy welcomed Kristy and treated her as their own grandchild. They adored her and treated her like the little princess she is. They loved to tell others about her. I feel that their love plus the love of my heavenly Father helped enable me to give so much love and care to little Kristy.

A Refuge for the Oppressed

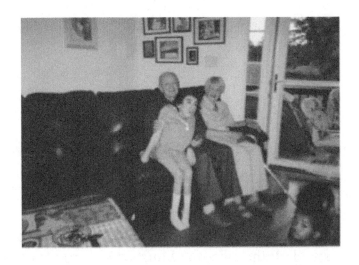

Missionaries to Paraguay
Blessed Kristy and praised her as an Inspiration

Psalm 9:9-10
The Lord also will be a refuge for the oppressed,
A refuge in the time of trouble
And those who know Your name will put their trust in You;
For You, Lord, have not forsaken those who seek You.

The afflicted are often oppressed in this world. How
comforting to know that God is with them. He is their
refuge and He will never forsake them.

Is There Not a Cause?

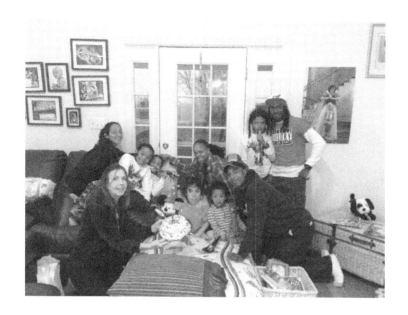

The Osborne Family Believed in God.
They were faithful friends, family to her and helped
Kristy from age 2.

Psalms 140:12 *I know the Lord will maintain the cause of the afflicted, and the right of the poor.*

Isaiah 63:9 *In all their affliction, He was afflicted. And the angel of His Presence saved them.*

Those who are afflicted have earnest cause. This verse provides comfort to anyone suffering because they are poor or afflicted. The Lord is on your side. He will maintain the cause so important to your life and heart. He will fight for you.

The battle is the Lord's.

God is Strength to the Poor, the Needy And Power to the Weak

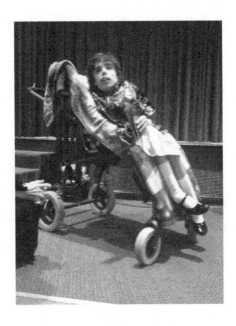

Isaiah 25:4 For You have been a strength to the poor, A strength to the needy in his distress, a refuge from the storm, a shade from the heat.

Isaiah 40: 27 – 29 Why do you say, O Jacob, And speak, O Israel: My way is hidden from the Lord, and my just claim is passed over by my God? Have you not known? Have you not heard? The everlasting God, the Lord, The Creator of the ends of the earth, neither faints nor is weary. There is no searching of His understanding. He gives power to the weak. And to those who have no might He increases strength.

The resource of God's strength and understanding is there in times of distress.

What do You Dream
When you Dream, Kristy?

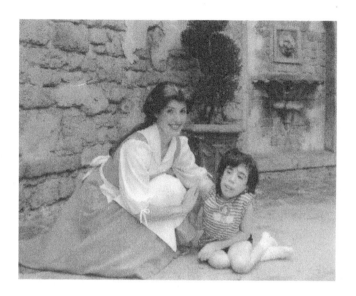

One prayer I prayed over and over with Kristy at her
bedside is that she would dream that she was walking and
talking, dancing, and running. I prayed that the dream
would be so real that she would feel that it was true.

Let us all pray for Kristy and all children and adults with
physical and mental challenges. Let us pray for miracles
that their dreams will come true. Let us also pray for
answers through medical research that cures will be found
and devices perfected to help and assist anyone suffering
disability.

I John 5:14 *This is the confidence we have in approaching
God: that if we ask anything according to His will, He hears
us.*

Treasures Awaiting in Heaven

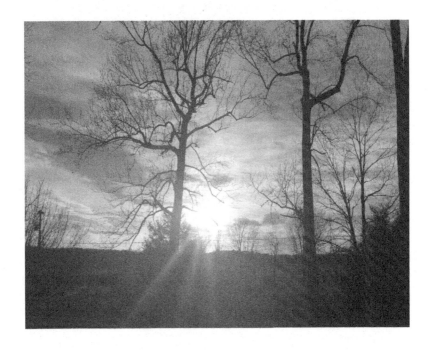

Isaiah 54:11 *O ye afflicted one, I will lay your stones with colorful gems and lay your foundations with sapphires.*

The Afflicted
Shall Eat at the King's Table

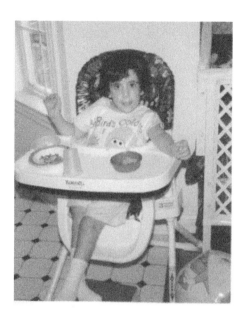

2 Samuel 9:1, 3, 5, 7
Now David said, "Is there still anyone who is left of the house of Saul that I may show kindness for Jonathan's sake?" And Ziba said, "There is still a son of Jonathan who is lame in his feet." Then King David sent and brought him out of the house of Machir, the son of Ammiel, from Lo Debar. So David said to him, "Do not fear, for I will surely show you kindness for Jonathan your father's sake, and will restore to you all the land of Saul your grandfather, and you shall eat bread at my tale continually."

Is the sweet story of King David's kindness to honor Mephibosheth but a looking glass into heaven and eternity where the King of Kings will bring the lame and afflicted to His great table?

Our Creator is Vigilant for the Weak

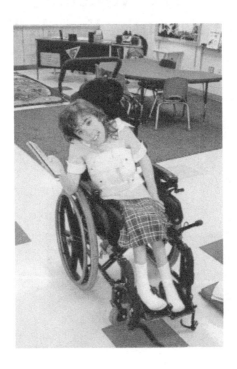

Isaiah 25:4 For You have been a strength to the poor, A strength to the needy in his distress, a refuge from the storm, a shade from the heat.

Isaiah 40: 27 – 29 Why do you say, O Jacob, And speak, O Israel: My way is hidden from the Lord, and my just claim is passed over by my God? Have you not known? Have you not heard? The everlasting God, the Lord, The Creator of the ends of the earth, neither faints nor is weary. There is no searching of His understanding. He gives power to the weak. And to those who have no might He increases strength.

The resource of God's strength and understanding is there in times of distress.

Kristy is in Everlasting Arms

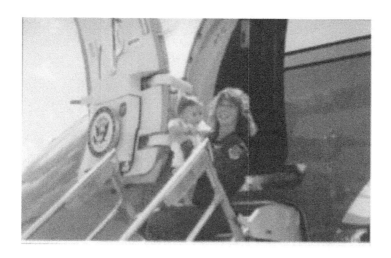

Deuteronomy 33:26-27
There is no one like the God of Jeshurun,
Who rides the heavens to help you
And in His Excellency on the clouds
The Eternal God is your refuge,
And underneath are the everlasting arms

As my arms have grown weaker and weaker from lifting Kristy all her life, it is comforting to know that she is in God's everlasting arms.

The First Shall be Last and the Last First

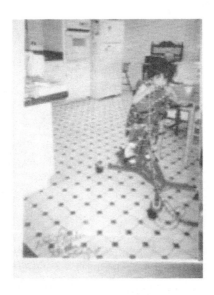

Luke 9:48 Prophetic words from Luke, a Physician, *For he who is least among you all will be great. For the first shall be last, and the last first.*

While the afflicted are often last and least in the world's eyes, so quickly discounted by harsh judgments of cruel self-righteousness or a materialistic society, they will be first in heaven and receive recognition and reward for all their sufferings.

There is exemplary greatness in their spirit in which they graciously bear their affliction, their courage engraved in eternal record.

Kristy's life is more important than mine. This truth became more and more evident in all the many trials we've suffered through throughout the years.

Help the Afflicted and
You Will Be Blessed

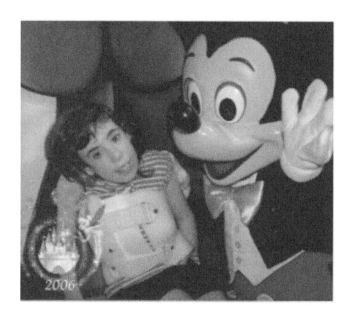

Mark 9:41
*For whoever gives you a cup of water to drink in
My name, because He belongs to Christ, I say to
you, he will by no means lose his reward.*

Life has proven this. Each one who has ever helped
the afflicted can testify that in so doing, blessing
has come. God's promise is sure that there is
reward for those who minister to others in His
name.

Job 6:14 *To him who is afflicted, kindness should be
shown by his friend.*

What Can I Do?

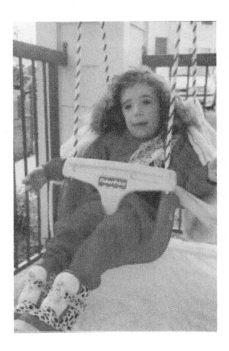

You may be wondering how you might help or what you can do? Begin with just a smile and say, "Hello."

So many people walk by or ignore persons with disabilities, even handicapped children. Little Kristy's eyes light up whenever anyone looks her in the eye, giving her attention and kindness or says her name, Kristy. Just saying hello and giving your name or calling theirs means so much to the person and to their family.

Remember, you too are a blessing from God and you bless others when you are kind.

Extraordinary, Dedicated Professionals
Who Contributed to Kristy's Life

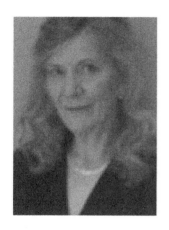 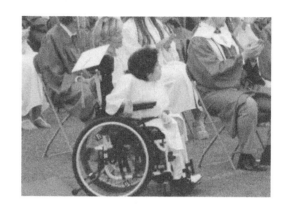

Dr. Margreete Johnston Mitzi Burton
Kristy's physician   High School
From birth   Special Ed Teacher

Prayer from the Depths
of the Soul of the Afflicted

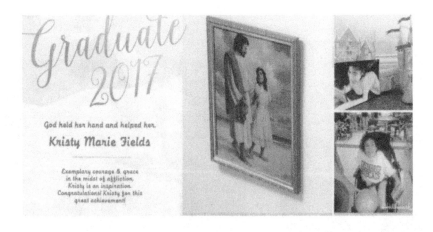

I believe God speaks, reveals Himself and His presence in a special way to those who are suffering and afflicted in this world. And I believe that prayers are lifted to heaven from the heart and souls of persons who may not be able to speak or verbalize the words of their most sincere cries, pleas, begging for mercy, for relief from pain and suffering, for help and deliverance. This relationship and communication between the Creator and His suffering child is so precious and special, a treasure of comfort for each one suffering.

Prayers are eternal and suffering as well is recorded in eternal record.

Psalms 90:15 *Make us glad according to the days in which You have afflicted us.*

Overcoming
To him that overcometh will I grant to sit with me in my throne

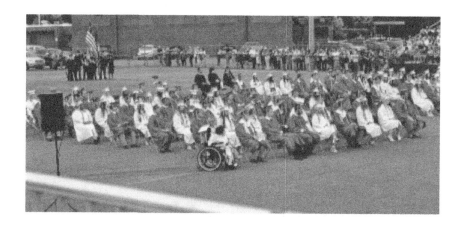

Greenbrier High School
Graduating Class of 2017

What a great day when little Kristy, who could not walk or talk, graduated from high school! She endured so much hardship through the years like riding a school bus through country roads in a wheelchair.

Oh! But what a blessing that she got to be with children her own age! She met so many wonderful people, the bus drivers, the school staff, the cafeteria workers, and the teachers who blessed her school days.

May God bless each one who blessed her.

Through the Waters

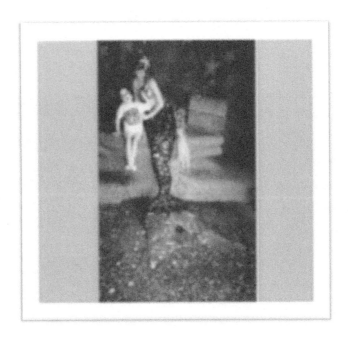

Isaiah 43
When you pass through the waters,
I will be with you.
And through the rivers,
They shall not overflow you.

How else did Kristy make it through all she has been through in her sweet life of many afflictions? God was and is with her.

Jesus Healed and Helped the Afflicted

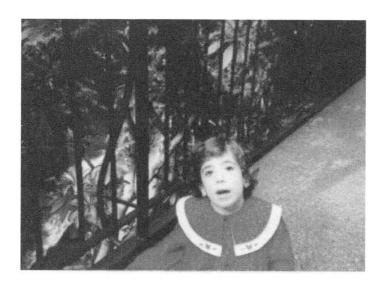

Matthew 4:23-24 *Now Jesus went about all Galilee, teaching in their synagogues, preaching the gospel of the kingdom, and healing all kinds of sickness and all kinds of disease among the people. And his fame went throughout all Syria; and they brought to Him all sick people who were afflicted with various diseases and torments, and those who were demon-possessed, epileptics, and paralytics; and He healed them.*

The Lame, the Infirm,
The One Sick of the Palsy

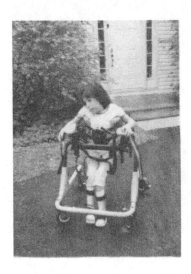

Mark 2:3 Jesus healed one sick of the palsy, carried by four friends who let him down through the roof. *I say to you, arise, take up your bed, and go your way to your house.*

Luke 13:11-12 *And behold, there was a woman who had a spirit of infirmity eighteen years, and was bent over and could in no way raise herself up. But when Jesus saw her, He called her to Him and said to her, Woman, you are loosed from your infirmity.*

John 5:2-9 Jesus healed the lame man at the Pool of Bethesda, by the Sheep Gate in Jerusalem. *Jesus said to him, Rise take up your bed and walk.*

Message of Hope and Heaven

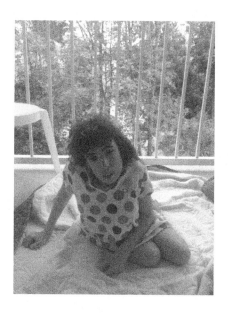

Hebrews 12:12-13 *Wherefore lift up the hands which hang down, and the palsied knees, and make straight paths for your feet, that that which is lame be not turned out of the way, but rather be healed.*

Revelation 2:9 *I know your works, tribulation, and poverty (but you are rich) . . .Be faithful until death and I will give you a crown of life.*

Revelation 21:4 *And God shall wipe away every tear from their eyes; there shall be no more death, nor sorrow, nor crying: and there shall be no more pain, for the former things have passed away.*

How Can a Little Girl Who Cannot Walk or Talk Be One the Bravest Person I Ever Met?

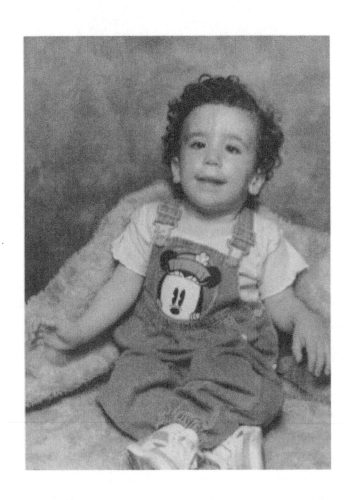

What a Blessing!
Brave, Smart, Little Crippled Angel

So Brave! Nursing in the some of the largest medical center emergency rooms in the country, Charity in New Orleans, Hermann (University of Texas Health Science Center), the Life Flight in Houston, Mt. Carmel and Detroit Receiving Hospital in Detroit, and Vanderbilt in Nashville, then on medical missions trips to China, Africa, India, Chile, Venezuela, Paraguay, Haiti, and Costa Rica, I've seen a lot of suffering. No one has been more brave in suffering than Kristy throughout many surgeries, illnesses, hospitalizations, and other afflictions and hardships. She has somehow managed a smile or a light pat on my back in her darkest and most difficult trials. I could not be more proud of her. She is one of the bravest people on the planet.

What does Kristy know? Kristy knows Jesus.

Although Kristy cannot walk or talk, she is fully aware of those in her life. I can just say certain names and she will smile or her eyes light up when I say the name of persons she knows. She certainly knows Jesus and when I say the name, Jesus, Kristy smiles and I see a light in her eyes like none other name I say. He is her friend and He is her Savior and she knows Him.

A Dream Come True

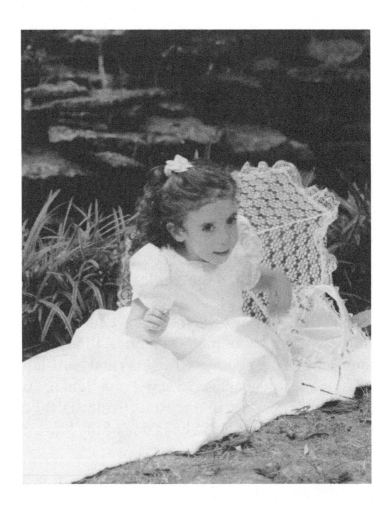

Before I ever met Kristy or she came to me, I dreamed of a little girl with thick dark brown curls.

The child in my dream was Kristy. I saw her before I ever met her.

A Song For Kristy

Don't worry little angel
God's watching over you

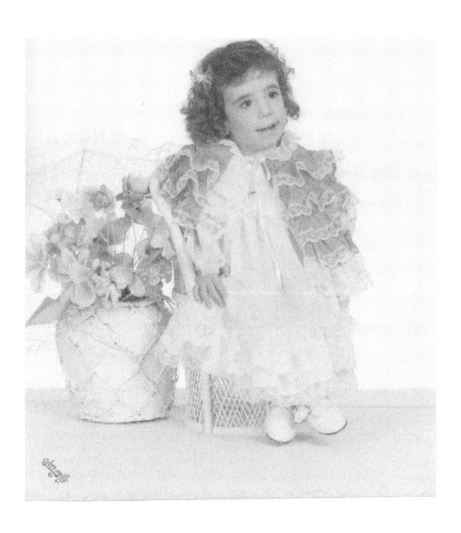

A Song for Kristy

No matter what troubles come
He will see you through.

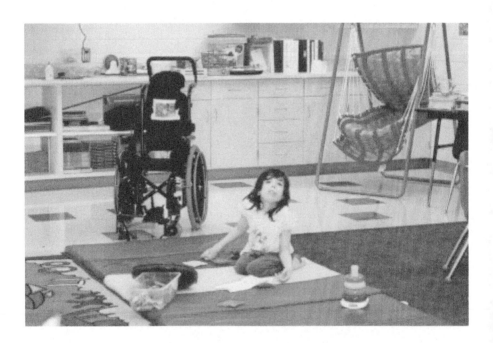

A Song for Kristy

He loves you, little angel,
You're ever in His care.

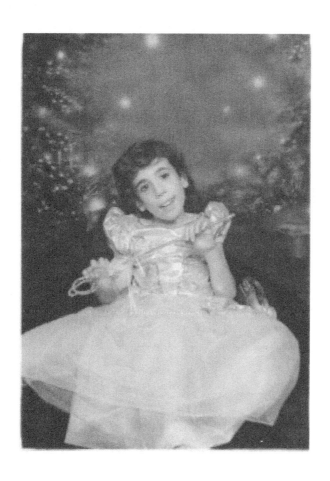

A Song for Kristy

Don't worry little angel,
God is always there.

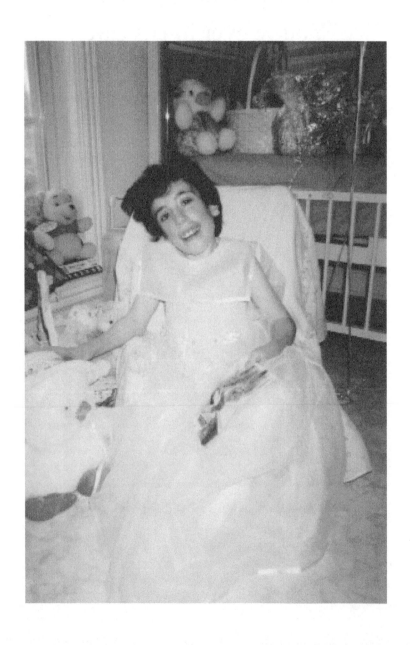

Angels Keep You

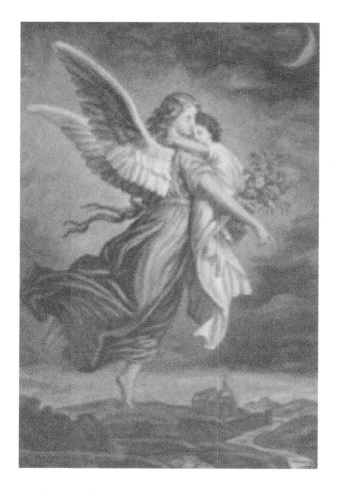

Image from greeting card sent to Kristy

Psalms 91
He shall give His Angels Charge over you to keep you in all your ways.
They shall bear you up lest you dash your foot against the stone. Amen

Only God Made This All Happen
To Him be the Glory

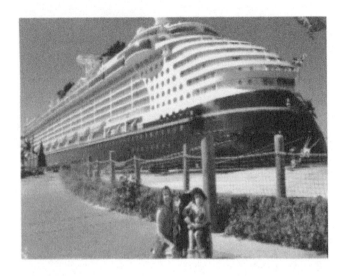

In the end, I know that God loved and helped Kristy through me. I am not that strong, or gifted, or good as I have been for Kristy. As I look back over the 23 years she has been in my care, I am amazed myself that we have made it. Most of her life, I worked 3 jobs, took care of a house and the yard while striving to fight a thousand battles for this little girl who was at death's door more times than I want to remember. Only God could have done this. He cared for Kristy through me and through many others. His care is excellent. I see His hand in all that has happened in Kristy's life. He is Kristy's Heavenly Father. She is God's child.

Miracle on My Street

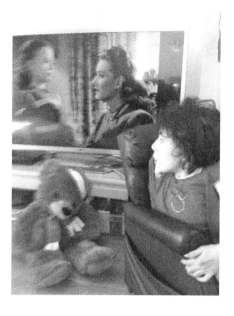

These few pictures and words fail to reveal the miraculous person that Kristy is. To God be the glory for sending His Son, Jesus, to die for Kristy and save her life, for one day in heaven Kristy will walk and talk.

Feeling God love her through me has been one of the very greatest blessings of my life.

Words cannot express such sweetness of God and of Kristy coming together. That I could be in this heaven and earth connection was transformational for me. And yes, I would do it again, a thousand times, yes! Amen.

Made in United States
Orlando, FL
24 January 2023

29002608R00032